Patient Registration Log

I0475179

DATE:

PATIENT NUMBER	PATIENT'S NAME	CONTACT NUMBER	TIME OF APPOINTMENT	TIME OF ARRIVAL

DATE:				
PATIENT NUMBER	PATIENT'S NAME	CONTACT NUMBER	TIME OF APPOINTMENT	TIME OF ARRIVAL

DATE:

PATIENT NUMBER	PATIENT'S NAME	CONTACT NUMBER	TIME OF APPOINTMENT	TIME OF ARRIVAL

DATE:

PATIENT NUMBER	PATIENT'S NAME	CONTACT NUMBER	TIME OF APPOINTMENT	TIME OF ARRIVAL

DATE:

PATIENT NUMBER	PATIENT'S NAME	CONTACT NUMBER	TIME OF APPOINTMENT	TIME OF ARRIVAL

DATE:

PATIENT NUMBER	PATIENT'S NAME	CONTACT NUMBER	TIME OF APPOINTMENT	TIME OF ARRIVAL

DATE:

PATIENT NUMBER	PATIENT'S NAME	CONTACT NUMBER	TIME OF APPOINTMENT	TIME OF ARRIVAL

DATE:

PATIENT NUMBER	PATIENT'S NAME	CONTACT NUMBER	TIME OF APPOINTMENT	TIME OF ARRIVAL

DATE:

PATIENT NUMBER	PATIENT'S NAME	CONTACT NUMBER	TIME OF APPOINTMENT	TIME OF ARRIVAL

DATE:

PATIENT NUMBER	PATIENT'S NAME	CONTACT NUMBER	TIME OF APPOINTMENT	TIME OF ARRIVAL

DATE:

PATIENT NUMBER	PATIENT'S NAME	CONTACT NUMBER	TIME OF APPOINTMENT	TIME OF ARRIVAL

DATE:

PATIENT NUMBER	PATIENT'S NAME	CONTACT NUMBER	TIME OF APPOINTMENT	TIME OF ARRIVAL

DATE:

PATIENT NUMBER	PATIENT'S NAME	CONTACT NUMBER	TIME OF APPOINTMENT	TIME OF ARRIVAL

DATE:

PATIENT NUMBER	PATIENT'S NAME	CONTACT NUMBER	TIME OF APPOINTMENT	TIME OF ARRIVAL

DATE:

PATIENT NUMBER	PATIENT'S NAME	CONTACT NUMBER	TIME OF APPOINTMENT	TIME OF ARRIVAL

DATE:

PATIENT NUMBER	PATIENT'S NAME	CONTACT NUMBER	TIME OF APPOINTMENT	TIME OF ARRIVAL

DATE:

PATIENT NUMBER	PATIENT'S NAME	CONTACT NUMBER	TIME OF APPOINTMENT	TIME OF ARRIVAL

DATE:

PATIENT NUMBER	PATIENT'S NAME	CONTACT NUMBER	TIME OF APPOINTMENT	TIME OF ARRIVAL

DATE:				
PATIENT NUMBER	PATIENT'S NAME	CONTACT NUMBER	TIME OF APPOINTMENT	TIME OF ARRIVAL

DATE:

PATIENT NUMBER	PATIENT'S NAME	CONTACT NUMBER	TIME OF APPOINTMENT	TIME OF ARRIVAL

DATE:

PATIENT NUMBER	PATIENT'S NAME	CONTACT NUMBER	TIME OF APPOINTMENT	TIME OF ARRIVAL

DATE:				
PATIENT NUMBER	PATIENT'S NAME	CONTACT NUMBER	TIME OF APPOINTMENT	TIME OF ARRIVAL

DATE:

PATIENT NUMBER	PATIENT'S NAME	CONTACT NUMBER	TIME OF APPOINTMENT	TIME OF ARRIVAL

DATE:

PATIENT NUMBER	PATIENT'S NAME	CONTACT NUMBER	TIME OF APPOINTMENT	TIME OF ARRIVAL

DATE:

PATIENT NUMBER	PATIENT'S NAME	CONTACT NUMBER	TIME OF APPOINTMENT	TIME OF ARRIVAL

DATE:

PATIENT NUMBER	PATIENT'S NAME	CONTACT NUMBER	TIME OF APPOINTMENT	TIME OF ARRIVAL

DATE:

PATIENT NUMBER	PATIENT'S NAME	CONTACT NUMBER	TIME OF APPOINTMENT	TIME OF ARRIVAL

DATE:

PATIENT NUMBER	PATIENT'S NAME	CONTACT NUMBER	TIME OF APPOINTMENT	TIME OF ARRIVAL

DATE:				
PATIENT NUMBER	PATIENT'S NAME	CONTACT NUMBER	TIME OF APPOINTMENT	TIME OF ARRIVAL

DATE:

PATIENT NUMBER	PATIENT'S NAME	CONTACT NUMBER	TIME OF APPOINTMENT	TIME OF ARRIVAL

DATE:

PATIENT NUMBER	PATIENT'S NAME	CONTACT NUMBER	TIME OF APPOINTMENT	TIME OF ARRIVAL

DATE:

PATIENT NUMBER	PATIENT'S NAME	CONTACT NUMBER	TIME OF APPOINTMENT	TIME OF ARRIVAL

DATE:

PATIENT NUMBER	PATIENT'S NAME	CONTACT NUMBER	TIME OF APPOINTMENT	TIME OF ARRIVAL

DATE:				
PATIENT NUMBER	PATIENT'S NAME	CONTACT NUMBER	TIME OF APPOINTMENT	TIME OF ARRIVAL

DATE:

PATIENT NUMBER	PATIENT'S NAME	CONTACT NUMBER	TIME OF APPOINTMENT	TIME OF ARRIVAL

DATE:

PATIENT NUMBER	PATIENT'S NAME	CONTACT NUMBER	TIME OF APPOINTMENT	TIME OF ARRIVAL

DATE:

PATIENT NUMBER	PATIENT'S NAME	CONTACT NUMBER	TIME OF APPOINTMENT	TIME OF ARRIVAL

DATE:

PATIENT NUMBER	PATIENT'S NAME	CONTACT NUMBER	TIME OF APPOINTMENT	TIME OF ARRIVAL

DATE:

PATIENT NUMBER	PATIENT'S NAME	CONTACT NUMBER	TIME OF APPOINTMENT	TIME OF ARRIVAL

DATE:

PATIENT NUMBER	PATIENT'S NAME	CONTACT NUMBER	TIME OF APPOINTMENT	TIME OF ARRIVAL

DATE:				
PATIENT NUMBER	PATIENT'S NAME	CONTACT NUMBER	TIME OF APPOINTMENT	TIME OF ARRIVAL

DATE:				
PATIENT NUMBER	PATIENT'S NAME	CONTACT NUMBER	TIME OF APPOINTMENT	TIME OF ARRIVAL

DATE:

PATIENT NUMBER	PATIENT'S NAME	CONTACT NUMBER	TIME OF APPOINTMENT	TIME OF ARRIVAL

DATE:

PATIENT NUMBER	PATIENT'S NAME	CONTACT NUMBER	TIME OF APPOINTMENT	TIME OF ARRIVAL

DATE:

PATIENT NUMBER	PATIENT'S NAME	CONTACT NUMBER	TIME OF APPOINTMENT	TIME OF ARRIVAL

DATE:				
PATIENT NUMBER	PATIENT'S NAME	CONTACT NUMBER	TIME OF APPOINTMENT	TIME OF ARRIVAL

DATE:

PATIENT NUMBER	PATIENT'S NAME	CONTACT NUMBER	TIME OF APPOINTMENT	TIME OF ARRIVAL

DATE:

PATIENT NUMBER	PATIENT'S NAME	CONTACT NUMBER	TIME OF APPOINTMENT	TIME OF ARRIVAL

DATE:

PATIENT NUMBER	PATIENT'S NAME	CONTACT NUMBER	TIME OF APPOINTMENT	TIME OF ARRIVAL

DATE:

PATIENT NUMBER	PATIENT'S NAME	CONTACT NUMBER	TIME OF APPOINTMENT	TIME OF ARRIVAL

DATE:

PATIENT NUMBER	PATIENT'S NAME	CONTACT NUMBER	TIME OF APPOINTMENT	TIME OF ARRIVAL

DATE:

PATIENT NUMBER	PATIENT'S NAME	CONTACT NUMBER	TIME OF APPOINTMENT	TIME OF ARRIVAL

DATE:

PATIENT NUMBER	PATIENT'S NAME	CONTACT NUMBER	TIME OF APPOINTMENT	TIME OF ARRIVAL

DATE:

PATIENT NUMBER	PATIENT'S NAME	CONTACT NUMBER	TIME OF APPOINTMENT	TIME OF ARRIVAL

DATE:

PATIENT NUMBER	PATIENT'S NAME	CONTACT NUMBER	TIME OF APPOINTMENT	TIME OF ARRIVAL

DATE:

PATIENT NUMBER	PATIENT'S NAME	CONTACT NUMBER	TIME OF APPOINTMENT	TIME OF ARRIVAL

DATE:				
PATIENT NUMBER	PATIENT'S NAME	CONTACT NUMBER	TIME OF APPOINTMENT	TIME OF ARRIVAL

DATE:

PATIENT NUMBER	PATIENT'S NAME	CONTACT NUMBER	TIME OF APPOINTMENT	TIME OF ARRIVAL

DATE:				
PATIENT NUMBER	PATIENT'S NAME	CONTACT NUMBER	TIME OF APPOINTMENT	TIME OF ARRIVAL

DATE:

PATIENT NUMBER	PATIENT'S NAME	CONTACT NUMBER	TIME OF APPOINTMENT	TIME OF ARRIVAL

DATE:

PATIENT NUMBER	PATIENT'S NAME	CONTACT NUMBER	TIME OF APPOINTMENT	TIME OF ARRIVAL

DATE:

PATIENT NUMBER	PATIENT'S NAME	CONTACT NUMBER	TIME OF APPOINTMENT	TIME OF ARRIVAL

DATE:				
PATIENT NUMBER	PATIENT'S NAME	CONTACT NUMBER	TIME OF APPOINTMENT	TIME OF ARRIVAL

DATE:

PATIENT NUMBER	PATIENT'S NAME	CONTACT NUMBER	TIME OF APPOINTMENT	TIME OF ARRIVAL

DATE:

PATIENT NUMBER	PATIENT'S NAME	CONTACT NUMBER	TIME OF APPOINTMENT	TIME OF ARRIVAL

DATE:

PATIENT NUMBER	PATIENT'S NAME	CONTACT NUMBER	TIME OF APPOINTMENT	TIME OF ARRIVAL

DATE:

PATIENT NUMBER	PATIENT'S NAME	CONTACT NUMBER	TIME OF APPOINTMENT	TIME OF ARRIVAL

DATE:

PATIENT NUMBER	PATIENT'S NAME	CONTACT NUMBER	TIME OF APPOINTMENT	TIME OF ARRIVAL

DATE:

PATIENT NUMBER	PATIENT'S NAME	CONTACT NUMBER	TIME OF APPOINTMENT	TIME OF ARRIVAL

DATE:

PATIENT NUMBER	PATIENT'S NAME	CONTACT NUMBER	TIME OF APPOINTMENT	TIME OF ARRIVAL

DATE:

PATIENT NUMBER	PATIENT'S NAME	CONTACT NUMBER	TIME OF APPOINTMENT	TIME OF ARRIVAL

DATE:

PATIENT NUMBER	PATIENT'S NAME	CONTACT NUMBER	TIME OF APPOINTMENT	TIME OF ARRIVAL

DATE:

PATIENT NUMBER	PATIENT'S NAME	CONTACT NUMBER	TIME OF APPOINTMENT	TIME OF ARRIVAL

DATE:

PATIENT NUMBER	PATIENT'S NAME	CONTACT NUMBER	TIME OF APPOINTMENT	TIME OF ARRIVAL

DATE:

PATIENT NUMBER	PATIENT'S NAME	CONTACT NUMBER	TIME OF APPOINTMENT	TIME OF ARRIVAL

DATE:

PATIENT NUMBER	PATIENT'S NAME	CONTACT NUMBER	TIME OF APPOINTMENT	TIME OF ARRIVAL

DATE:

PATIENT NUMBER	PATIENT'S NAME	CONTACT NUMBER	TIME OF APPOINTMENT	TIME OF ARRIVAL

DATE:

PATIENT NUMBER	PATIENT'S NAME	CONTACT NUMBER	TIME OF APPOINTMENT	TIME OF ARRIVAL

DATE:

PATIENT NUMBER	PATIENT'S NAME	CONTACT NUMBER	TIME OF APPOINTMENT	TIME OF ARRIVAL

DATE:

PATIENT NUMBER	PATIENT'S NAME	CONTACT NUMBER	TIME OF APPOINTMENT	TIME OF ARRIVAL

DATE:

PATIENT NUMBER	PATIENT'S NAME	CONTACT NUMBER	TIME OF APPOINTMENT	TIME OF ARRIVAL

DATE:

PATIENT NUMBER	PATIENT'S NAME	CONTACT NUMBER	TIME OF APPOINTMENT	TIME OF ARRIVAL

DATE:

PATIENT NUMBER	PATIENT'S NAME	CONTACT NUMBER	TIME OF APPOINTMENT	TIME OF ARRIVAL

DATE:

PATIENT NUMBER	PATIENT'S NAME	CONTACT NUMBER	TIME OF APPOINTMENT	TIME OF ARRIVAL

DATE:

PATIENT NUMBER	PATIENT'S NAME	CONTACT NUMBER	TIME OF APPOINTMENT	TIME OF ARRIVAL

DATE:

PATIENT NUMBER	PATIENT'S NAME	CONTACT NUMBER	TIME OF APPOINTMENT	TIME OF ARRIVAL

DATE:

PATIENT NUMBER	PATIENT'S NAME	CONTACT NUMBER	TIME OF APPOINTMENT	TIME OF ARRIVAL

DATE:

PATIENT NUMBER	PATIENT'S NAME	CONTACT NUMBER	TIME OF APPOINTMENT	TIME OF ARRIVAL

DATE:

PATIENT NUMBER	PATIENT'S NAME	CONTACT NUMBER	TIME OF APPOINTMENT	TIME OF ARRIVAL

DATE:

PATIENT NUMBER	PATIENT'S NAME	CONTACT NUMBER	TIME OF APPOINTMENT	TIME OF ARRIVAL

DATE:				
PATIENT NUMBER	PATIENT'S NAME	CONTACT NUMBER	TIME OF APPOINTMENT	TIME OF ARRIVAL

DATE:				
PATIENT NUMBER	PATIENT'S NAME	CONTACT NUMBER	TIME OF APPOINTMENT	TIME OF ARRIVAL

DATE:

PATIENT NUMBER	PATIENT'S NAME	CONTACT NUMBER	TIME OF APPOINTMENT	TIME OF ARRIVAL

DATE:

PATIENT NUMBER	PATIENT'S NAME	CONTACT NUMBER	TIME OF APPOINTMENT	TIME OF ARRIVAL

DATE:

PATIENT NUMBER	PATIENT'S NAME	CONTACT NUMBER	TIME OF APPOINTMENT	TIME OF ARRIVAL

DATE:

PATIENT NUMBER	PATIENT'S NAME	CONTACT NUMBER	TIME OF APPOINTMENT	TIME OF ARRIVAL

DATE:				
PATIENT NUMBER	PATIENT'S NAME	CONTACT NUMBER	TIME OF APPOINTMENT	TIME OF ARRIVAL

DATE:

PATIENT NUMBER	PATIENT'S NAME	CONTACT NUMBER	TIME OF APPOINTMENT	TIME OF ARRIVAL

DATE:

PATIENT NUMBER	PATIENT'S NAME	CONTACT NUMBER	TIME OF APPOINTMENT	TIME OF ARRIVAL

www.ingramcontent.com/pod-product-compliance
Lightning Source LLC
Chambersburg PA
CBHW081827170526
45167CB00007B/2740
* 9 7 8 1 5 4 2 8 6 4 6 9 5 *